Is Acupuncture for You?

Is

ACUPUNCTURE

FOR YOU?

J. R. WORSLEY

President, College of Chinese Acupuncture (U.K.)
Professor, Chinese College of Acupuncture (China)
Master and Doctor of Acupuncture (China)

HARPER & ROW, PUBLISHERS
New York • Evanston • San Francisco • London

Portions of chapter 12, "Soviet and Korean Research Substantiating Acupuncture," have appeared in *Galaxies of Life*, edited by Stanley Krippner and Daniel Rubin (New York: Gordon and Breach, 1973).

Designed by C. Linda Dingler

Library of Congress Cataloging in Publication Data

Worsley, J R
  Is acupuncture for you?

  1. Acupuncture. I. Title. [DNLM: 1. Acupuncture. WB 369 W931i 1973]
RM184.W67 1973   615'.89   72-9874
ISBN 0-06-069690-7
ISBN 0-06-069691-5 (pbk)

Contents

Illustrations appear on pages 5, 9, 11, 19 and 48

Foreword

by The Rt. Rev. The Lord Bishop of Coventry

The reader may wonder why I, who know little about acupuncture, am writing this foreword. I am doing so because I feel it is important that in the closely knit world of today we, in the West, should not cling determinedly to the ideas and practices of the West alone, but that we should be willing to approach valued ideas from other parts of the world with open minds and a willingness to learn.

We cannot afford to ignore or wave aside any method of helping mankind simply because it sounds at first to our Western ears a little odd or even incredible.

I have been impressed by what I have heard about acupuncture; the breadth of its approach to the health of the whole person—body, mind and spirit; and the importance that it places upon the way of life that we choose to lead.

This little book should be of great interest to many and I commend it to you.

CUTHBERT COVENTRY

Bishop's House, Coventry, England

Preface

With the gentle raising of the bamboo curtain, increasing reports to the American public from the People's Republic of China are filtering through the press which are short of staggering to the human mind. In fact, since President Richard Nixon's visit to China in late February, 1972, highlighted by demonstrations of acupuncture anesthesia and succeeding T.V. programs, acupuncture has become virtually a household word.

Certainly 5,000 years of continuous and successful use of this art can hardly be set aside by cries of hypnotism, suggestion, psychosomatics, lack of scientific evidence, and quackery. Call it what you will, but no one can deny that acupuncture has stunned this nation with its use in anesthesia, control of pain, and a miscellany of problems long defiant of medical practice such as arthritis, deafness, paralysis, migraine, et al. There are few who would not be willing to climb upon the bandwagon— either to administer or receive—so fascinating does this subject impress the vision and mind.

China currently has 1,000,000 specialists trained in this field, of which 150,000 are physicians. Japan has 50,000, with perhaps 2,000 to 3,000 scattered throughout the western world, primarily in France, West Germany, Russia, Switzerland, and

England. There is but a handful in the United States primarily because a medical license is required here as in France.

Worsley has made a tremendous contribution in this little book which is written in a simple, readily understandable question-answer style. It answers any and all questions an inquisitive public might present to the master either during a personal interview or preparatory to actual treatment.

Worsley's other great legacy has been in the field of teaching. Founding the Chinese College of Acupuncture in England in 1960, he has trained countless eager students throughout the world in the intervening years. Occasional seminars have been given in the United States for the past two years, with the first full-month intensified course for Americans being completed in England in October, 1972. It is anticipated that this group, after additional study, will form the nucleus of an American College of Chinese Medicine.

As a practicing neurosurgeon for over twenty-five years, I have become increasingly disenchanted with the standard treatment of intractable pain, trigeminal neuralgia, neuritis, migraine, paralysis, and many other neurological problems.

It was only natural that I should be attracted to acupuncture in an effort to relieve further the sufferings of mankind. Worsley is a great teacher and clinician. This I can attest by personal experience. He is most able to tell us about the relationship of traditional Chinese medicine, including acupuncture, moxa, herbs, and physical therapy, to the Chinese philosophy of Taoism and the Yin-Yang concept of dynamically opposing, yet harmonizing forces in the universe.

William G. Peacher, M.D.

Attending Neurosurgeon
St. Joseph's Hospital
Syracuse, New York

Introduction

The first thing that struck me about J. R. Worsley when I met him was that he was everything I expected a doctor to be. He was thorough and efficient. He seemed to know what he was doing and was genuinely concerned about my welfare. The only question was whether he could help me, or had I come 4,000 costly miles from New York to England on some kind of wild goose chase?

A friend had recommended Worsley to me, and, although entirely coincidentally, he had appeared on a television program on the New York station for which I work. On the program, he had discussed the philosophy and history of acupuncture and had demonstrated a "typical" examination and treatment on a young patient and associate. That was the first time I had heard of the preventative and curative powers of acupuncture. Everything I had read up to that time stressed only the potential use and relatively recent development of acupuncture as an anesthetic. I was impressed by his presentation, but also very skeptical about his claims. Perhaps it was the television format which bothered me; but more likely, it was that he was asking me to accept a totally new form of treatment and a profoundly different philosophy of medicine.

Two months later I was in his office in England. I was there because two years before I had broken my neck in a freak surfing accident, and had suffered severe spinal damage. For almost three weeks I was totally paralyzed from my chest down. Miraculously, I had recovered. Although I was walking with the aid of a cane and was back at work, I still had major residual effects.

All the specialists I had seen said there was nothing they could do for me, that nature would have to take its course. And, they couldn't tell me whether I would ever recover more than I had already. I went to see Worsley because, I reasoned, I had nothing to lose but time and money. Also, I realized that it was not necessary for me to understand how acupuncture worked, if it worked, as I didn't understand how penicillin or aspirin worked and yet I had no hesitation about taking them. Since Worsley's appearance on television, I did some investigations of my own and satisfied myself that he was highly respected in the field and, further, that there was a considerable body of unpublicized evidence which claimed that acupuncture was in fact a very effective ancient art of healing.

It took Worsley about one and a half hours to give me the same thorough examination that he describes in this book. He then gave me a diagnosis and said it would take him another four to six hours to work out a plan of treatment. He said he thought he could help me, although he shared the same beliefs of my American doctors that if nerves had been totally destroyed, there was nothing to be done and that my "cure" was basically up to nature. The only difference was that Worsley felt acupuncture could help nature.

Back at our hotel, my wife and I discussed whether we should go ahead. We finally decided that we'd come too far to turn back and, more important, that I couldn't afford to turn my back on the only doctor who said he thought he could help me. Worsley gave me six treatments. Some of the results, though exciting, were only temporary. I found that for a short time after the second treatment and every treatment thereafter, I was free of the spasticity which plagued me by making movement extremely awkward and difficult. Most important, those six treatments succeeded in returning my bladder control to near normal. There were other things: I have very little sensation in my left leg and cannot feel pain or temperature. After one treatment with needles and moxa, I was, for a short time, able to feel pain.

I was most skeptical about how much Worsley could tell from my Chinese pulses—("What do you mean six pulses in each wrist? Everyone knows there is only one?") Yet, one day he correctly diagnosed and treated an upset stomach, cramps and diarrhea, which he had no way of knowing existed before he took my pulses.

I realize that all of this is anecdotal and far from scientific. However, all any layman can do is to report results. At the same time that we invited Dr. Worsley to appear on television, we also invited a number of prominent New York physicians who had recently been to China and had witnessed some forms of acupuncture. None of them would appear on the show with Worsley. It would seem to me that the intelligent thing for these gentlemen to do would be to talk with Worsley, to question him, to try to understand, to listen and to learn. Isn't it possible that this ancient form of medicine could be as helpful to us as it has been to the Chinese? I still don't fully understand how acupuncture works, but in my case, I know it worked.

JACK WILLIS

New York City

Author's Note

Acupuncture has attracted much attention in the West during the last few years. On many occasions it has been presented to the public as a panacea. Glowing reports have been made of its wonder cures. This can be damaging to acupuncture. I believe acupuncture to be one of the most wonderful systems of healing that there is and one that has truly stood the test of time, but like all other systems of healing, it has certain limitations. These are few, but it must nevertheless be emphasized that acupuncture is not a cure for everything. Furthermore, the results achieved will depend upon the training, skill, and experience of the practitioner.

In view of the uncertainty and confusion about acupuncture caused by conflicting reports, a number of American doctors, psychiatrists, and psychologists have approached me with the suggestion that in view of my long experience in the practice of and in teaching acupuncture, I should write a book for the American public to explain this method of healing. The present small volume is the result.

When people have been to me for treatment, they have usually wanted to know certain basic facts about how acupuncture works. Most people ask similar questions about the actual treatment, the illnesses that can be helped, the length of time it will take to regain health, and so on. The book is therefore presented in a question-and-answer form and follows through as a conversation between a questioner and myself.

The latter part of the book is concerned with our life-style in the West and the causative factors of disease. While it is true that we, as individuals, cannot change many of the things discussed, we should be aware of the stresses to which our way of life subjects us. If we are to maintain our health it is most important that each of us should individually adjust our way of living as far as possible to eliminate or lessen these stresses. Acupuncture can do much to help fight and prevent disease, but maintaining health is not the sole responsibility of the doctor; for the most part it is your own.

J. R. Worsley, Dr. Ac.

1.

What Is Acupuncture?

What is Acupuncture?

Acupuncture is one of the oldest forms of healing known to mankind. It originated in China nearly five thousand years ago. The fact that it is still being practised today, thousands of years later, speaks much for the efficacy of this treatment and for the laws and principles on which it is based. These are the laws and principles of all creation and they underlie the whole of Chinese culture, including all Chinese medical thinking.

Their application to the health of the human body was first written down about 400 B.C., a golden age of Chinese thought, in a book that remains the foundation of all Chinese medicine, of which acupuncture is an important part. This book, the *Nei Ching (The Yellow Emperor's Classic of Internal Medicine)*, is a treatise on life itself. As well as explaining how to live one's life in accordance with the great natural laws of the universe, and examining at length the normal functions of the human body, and bodily diseases and their causes, this book sets out for the first time a theory on which the whole of acupuncture is based. This is the meridian theory and is about the flow of life energy through a person's body. (I will discuss this in Chapters 3 and 12.)

Acupuncture treatment is usually carried out by inserting very fine needles into specific points on the body. The use of needles was introduced at about the same time as the writing of the *Nei Ching,* about 400 B.C.

Throughout this book when I speak of acupuncture I will mean traditional Chinese acupuncture. This is an art that takes a considerable number of years to learn and many, many more to gain the expertise of a master.

As can be imagined, there were many people in China who, without special study, picked up a little knowledge about acupuncture. They would notice that a particular treatment would be effective for relieving pain, and that another helped colic, and so on. And so there grew up the practice of treating one's family or local community for minor ailments. Anyone practicing in this way was known as a "local doctor" or "barefoot doctor". Valuable as this was in China's vast rural communities, it was not the traditional acupuncture. It was regarded rather as an emergency or first-aid service. The local doctor was treating quite specifically a symptom and was not seeking to remove the cause of the trouble, as does the traditional doctor.

This type of acupuncture is still practiced, and quite frequently in the West. The practitioner does not need such a lengthy training for this as he will be able to improve a symptom of illness long before he is skilled enough to remove the cause of it. This work is of course good in its place, but should not be confused with the wider aims of traditional acupuncture and should be viewed with caution by the seriously ill.

There is also the special use of acupuncture for anesthesia. This is much talked about in the West just now as the methods used are relatively new and are being much publicized by China. But this is something quite distinct from traditional acupuncture and is not really part of the work of the traditional doctor.

The practitioner of traditional Chinese acupuncture has

three aims in mind whenever he treats a patient. These are:

(1) To treat the patient as a whole.

This means he must consider the physical body and the mind together as one unity (referred to in this book as body +mind), and he must consider this unity as a part of the whole creation, having its own unique relationship with its environment.

(2) To seek for the cause of disease.

It is most important that he should not concern himself with the complaint itself, for this is only a symptom of disease in the body. He must always try to find the reason for this disease.

(3) Having found the cause, to attempt to remove it.

Once the trouble has been put right at its root, the symptoms of illness will disappear of themselves.

The doctor of acupuncture must strive to see his patient not as he is at the time of examination but as he would be if he were whole and perfect in body, mind, and spirit, with every possibility of his "unique being" realized. The personality and behavior of a person when ill will not necessarily be true to his own real nature, and may indeed be very different. The work of the doctor of traditional Chinese acupuncture is to help this sick person become renewed, revitalized, and brought to the fullness of his potential.

2.

The Use of Needles

Is anything in or on the needles?

No. The needles are solid stainless steel not much thicker than the hair on your head. No drugs of any kind are injected and there is no electric charge or current.

Does it hurt?

No. In some cases the needles can hardly be felt at all. Sometimes there will be a slight sensation of heat or numbness and occasionally a sharp prick, but these sensations are only momentary. In fact, it is much less painful than when you accidentally stick a pin or needle in yourself.

How would the insertion of an acupuncture needle compare with a western injection?

It is far less unpleasant. There is really no comparison. There are in fact many occasions when the patient is quite unaware that needles have been inserted.

How long are the needles? Do the length and style of the needles vary?

Yes, they vary in length from one-half inch to four inches. As you can see in the photograph, there are different types of needles. These will be used according to the effect that the practitioner wants to achieve. Some of these needles are specially made to be used in conjunction with moxa.

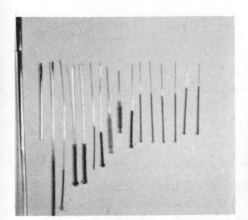 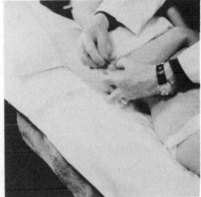

How deep are the needles inserted?

The depth of the insertion of the needle varies considerably and this depends on the point being used. Most needles are inserted just below the surface of the skin, but some may go from a depth of a quarter inch to as much as three inches. Do not be misled into thinking that the deeper the insertion, the more pain the patient feels. The patient may feel no more discomfort from a needle inserted three inches below the skin than from a needle inserted just below the skin.

Does the patient bleed very much?

Not at all. The actual points used do not bleed. However on occasions the practitioner may purposely bleed a point. The result of this would still only be one, two, or at the most three drops of blood.

Has a needle ever broken or bent during treatment?

The handmade Chinese needles that I use are pliable and it would be impossible to break them in use. They do sometimes bend slightly if the patient moves vigorously after the needle has been inserted. I am aware that there are some needles that possibly could break, but every fully qualified practitioner whom I have taught realizes the importance of the quality of needles and uses a reliable type.

Is the needle manipulated in any way after insertion?

This depends upon the effect desired. In some cases once the needle has been inserted it is not manipulated at all. In other cases it is manipulated in one of a number of different ways. For instance, many people will have heard of the twirling of a needle used for anesthesia.

Are the needles sterilized before treatment?

Yes. It is a fundamental practice to sterilize all needles.

Into what parts of the body does the acupuncturist insert the needles?

The part of the body into which one puts the needles usually bears no relation to the site of the disease or of the symptoms. The lower legs, the feet, the forearms, and the hands are the parts most frequently used, but the needles may be applied to any other part of the body.

How many needles are used?

This varies from one patient to another, but usually from three to eight would be used.

Have I heard something about gold and silver needles sometimes being used?

You may well have. This idea has probably arisen from mistakes made in translating the Chinese texts. The needles themselves were always made from the finest metal, but they were mounted either with gold or with silver according to whether they were being used on the mandarin classes or on the common people.

Are the needles made only in China? Are they manufactured by traditional or modern methods?

Needles are manufactured in many countries throughout the world, but I personally use Chinese needles that are handmade.

In the West there is an inclination to attach too much importance to the needle itself. It is the treatment and the particular point treated that matter. The effect of the treatment is not due to the metal or material of the needle. In China, acupuncture treatment was being given successfully long before metal needles were made, using needles made of bone.

The thing that we are really concerned with today is the quality of the needle and that it should be unbreakable.

3.

How It Works

Why does it work?

Acupuncture sets out to correct any imbalance that is in the body or in the mind and to restore harmony and equilibrium, thus eradicating the causative factors of sickness. If all of the functions and organs of the body are working properly and in harmony, then there cannot be sickness within the body or mind.

How can the acupuncturist bring about this balance in the body by inserting needles into it?

Traditional Chinese medicine states that the vital force, or life force, in the body controls the working of the main organs and systems of the body. This vital force, or Ch'i energy as it is called, circulates from one organ to another along channels or pathways termed meridians, always following a set route. This energy must flow freely in the correct strength and quality if each organ is to function correctly. In all illness the flow of vital energy is impaired. Whatever system of medicine is used to heal a patient, its success depends on the restoration of this vital force, Ch'i (pronounced *Kee*).

Acupuncture directly controls this energy at special points located on the meridians (the energy pathways). When gently inserted into these acupuncture points the needles produce various effects. According to the manipulation of the needles, the energy is either drawn to an organ, or dispersed from it, or drained, and so on.

The patient is sometimes able to observe this Ch'i energy at work by watching the movements of the needles. Sometimes they will be seen to vibrate for some considerable time while the flow of energy is being regulated. There are occasions when the energy grips the needle and holds it firmly until a balance has been reached in the Ch'i energy passing through that particular meridian. It would not be possible to remove this needle until a balance is reached, but as soon as its work is done it may fall out of its own accord. Very often when excess energy is being dispersed from a meridian the needle will drop out when the correct tension is restored.

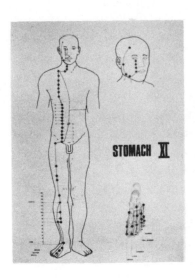

STOMACH II

4·

The Use of Moxa and Other Treatments

Does the practitioner use anything other than the needles?

Yes. And in some cases no needles at all are used. A special form of massage may be used on the acupuncture points, or the points may be heated in various ways. Sometimes a system of Chinese osteopathy is practiced.

How is the heat applied to the acupuncture points?

The usual way to heat an acupoint is for a tiny cone of moxa to be placed on the skin and ignited. Moxa is made from the herb *Artemisia vulgaris latiflora* and is rather like a brown-colored wool. The acupoint is heated deeply by this method. The moxa may be burnt on a bed of ginger, garlic, or salt to produce special effects. Alternatively, an area may be heated by a large burning moxa stick, three quarters of an inch to one and a half inches in diameter, which is passed backward and forward over the skin just close enough to give a comfortable heat. Moxa is also used on the head of special needles and ignited.

These are just a few of the ways that moxa may be used; the

method selected depends on what the practitioner wants to achieve.

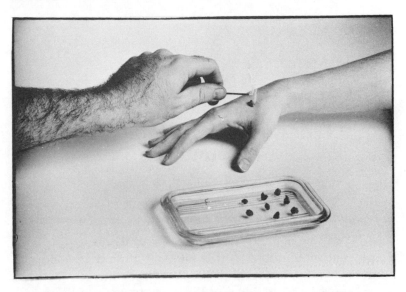

Does the moxa ever burn the skin?

No. It is removed when the patient feels sufficient heat. It is not left on the skin long enough to cause a burn, and if the treatment is carried out correctly there is no scar.

What is the difference between using moxa and using needles?

In some cases the insertion of needles may not be the appropriate technique, because of either the condition of the patient or the nature of the disease. For example, moxa may be particularly effective for treating certain cases of rheumatism, bone diseases, and cramps.

5.

Types of Illness Helped by Acupuncture

Is acupuncture helpful only for certain types of illness?

No. It can be applied successfully to all illness and in both simple and acute disorders it is safe and often dramatic in its effect. It is a fundamental principle of acupuncture that one should treat the body and mind as a whole, not just the symptom or the named disease. The practitioner must look for the cause of the disease and not for its manifestation; he must therefore ascertain the source of imbalance in the functioning of the body. There exist in the body twelve main organs and functions. All sickness is the result of the disordered working of one or more of these main organs and functions.

What about chronic illness? Could disease have gone too far for acupuncture to be able to help?

A time does come when disease is so deeply seated that the sufferer is beyond human help. But at all prior stages acupuncture can treat illness successfully. The treatment of the early stages is frequently dramatic, but if these early stages have been untreated or unsatisfactorily treated they will in the course of time cause organic change, and the simple illness becomes chronic. In this case, long and patient work by the doctor of acupuncture will be required.

In what cases would you definitely not recommend acupuncture treatment?

I would not recommend acupuncture treatment in those emergency cases resulting from accident or advanced disease where immediate surgical or medical treatment is needed to save the patient's life. There are also the terminal cases that I have already mentioned where the patient is beyond human help. Nevertheless, in such a case a decision might be reached to use acupuncture simply to relieve pain and suffering.

There are, however, cases in which a decision is difficult to reach. Consequently in every case, after examining the patient, I ask myself whether or not acupuncture is the best form of treatment for him. For a number of reasons it might be better to recommend treatment by orthodox medicine, surgery, and so on. In all cases of doubt my guideline is to ask myself what I would recommend if the patient were my wife, my son, my daughter, and so on.

Many people who are chronically ill must be under drugs constantly for various reasons including the relief of pain. Does this make the treatment of the illness more difficult?

It certainly doesn't make the practitioner's task any easier. Drugs may bring great relief to many sufferers but in the long run they harm the body and introduce something further for it to battle with. They tend to suppress the trouble rather than to remove the cause of it.

The healthy body itself makes all the drugs that it needs to fight disease, repair damage, and keep itself fit. The sick body does not do so. Acupuncture treatment aims to restore the body's own ability to produce the necessary enzymes and secretions: insulin, pepsin, adrenalin, cortisone, hydrochloric acid, and the like.

Does this mean that acupuncture can cure deficiency diseases?

In many cases deficiency diseases respond well to acupuncture treatment. In the West we tend to think that if the patient is deficient in a substance, we can cure him by dosing him with the substance concerned. We give him iron for anemia, insulin for diabetes, vitamins, calcium, hormones, and so on. The introduction of these substances does not usually correct the condition permanently; it only keeps the body going. The doctor of acupuncture aims to correct the cause of the deficiency, thus enabling the body to produce the necessary substances and to extract what is required from the normal diet.

Can acupuncture help in cases of addiction—drugs, alcohol, or even smoking?

Yes, it can help. A person who is perfectly healthy in body and in mind does not need the comfort, help, or stimulus of drugs or alcohol. Addiction to any of these is a sign of insecurity, stress, or strain, all of which are difficult to avoid in modern living. Acupuncture can correct the imbalance that has resulted but a permanent cure depends upon the removal or resolution of the stresses that caused the addiction.

Can acupuncture treatment be used during pregnancy?

Yes, it can, but it should be administered only by a highly qualified practitioner with long experience. Such a practitioner could safely treat many different illnesses while the patient was pregnant. Apart from illness, a skilled practitioner can certainly help to ensure that a pregnancy is a healthy one. In countless cases that I have treated the result has been a very healthy pregnancy, free from morning sickness, overweight problems, depression, and so on. In the final month of pregnancy the treatments given facilitate an easy, natural childbirth. In China they are using acupuncture anesthesia for childbirth with success.

Is acupuncture used for birth control and abortion?

In some eastern countries acupuncture has been used for both birth control and abortion. But this would never be carried out by a registered, qualified practitioner who had been trained by myself, as this is, for various practical and philosophical reasons, a violation of the code of ethics.

Does acupuncture aid the healing of broken bones?

Yes. The patient will still need to have the bone set in the usual way but acupuncture can assist and speed up the healing process. I have had cases where it has been possible for the cast to be removed some three weeks before it would normally be due to come off.

One of the most successful combinations of modern medicine and traditional Chinese acupuncture has taken place in this field in China. The Chinese claim to have shortened considerably the time taken to heal the fracture by dispensing with the cast and using thin splints that, while holding the bone firmly in position, allow a certain freedom of movement in the area. Acupuncture, by bringing energy to the area, helps to keep all the normal processes of that area of the body functioning fully, so leading to rapid healing.

Is acupuncture used to treat tumors?

The traditional Chinese acupuncturist does not treat named symptoms, and a tumor would come into this category. There are many recorded cases where tumors have disappeared during treatment, but others where treatment has been of no use whatsoever. So much depends on the causative factors of the disease and how far it has gone.

What about things like hay fever and other allergies and insomnia? Can it help here?

Hay fever and insomnia are again the names of symptoms. The causative factors of allergies and of insomnia can be numerous. They can result from tension, worry, fear, depression, grief, and many other mental factors; or they can result from organic malfunction; or in many cases they come from a combination of mental and organic factors. The hay fever and insomnia will clear up as the Ch'i energy in the patient is brought into balance.

Does this mean that mental illness comes within the scope of acupuncture?

Yes, indeed. I cannot stress too strongly that the doctor of acupuncture always views the body + mind as a whole. There is no division. All physical disorders will cause an imbalance in the mental outlook of a person. This may manifest itself as depression, anger, sadness, or the like. And all mental disturbances will cause some reaction in the physical body, such as sickness, insomnia, lack of appetite, weariness, and aching limbs. It is a two-way reaction: one cannot have a physical illness on its own, or a mental disturbance on its own. Any imbalance in a person must manifest itself both in the physical body and in the mental body, two parts of the one whole.

All treatments aim to restore the harmony of the body + mind and so the physical and mental sides of a person are treated together. As one improves, so does the other.

We hear a lot today about many illnesses being psychosomatic. You don't completely agree with this, then?

I would direct attention again to the two-way reaction between the physical body and the mind. Suppose a person were suffering from acute depression. This could be the manifestation of either mental difficulties or of a particular physical disorder, for example, malfunction of the kidneys or the bladder, or of any one or perhaps more of the other organs. It is extremely important to diagnose the cause of illness accurately in a case like this before treatment is given.

One of my patients came to me to be treated for lumbago. When she was better and had finished treatment her husband came to me and thanked me, not for curing her lumbago but for making his life so much happier again. Ilis wife had previously been so exceedingly irritable that she had been very difficult to live with. He had no idea when he offered to pay for her treatment that it was going to make such a change in her whole outlook. Now she was a happy cheerful person.

It does seem that western medicine does not always appreciate the effect that a physical disorder has on the mental state of a person. Each main organ and function has its counterpart in the mind, and the disordered working of each of these main organs and functions has a particular and different effect on the mental state of a person. These different mental states actually help the doctor of acupuncture to determine the source of disordered working in the physical body.

Will acupuncture benefit someone who is very skeptical?

Yes, certainly. The healing process will not be affected in any way by the patient's skeptical attitude.

6.

The Acupuncture Practitioner's Methods of Diagnosis

Does the acupuncture practitioner use different methods of diagnosis from those normally used by the Western doctor?

The methods of Chinese diagnosis are completely different from those we are accustomed to use in the West.

The ability of a skilled doctor of acupuncture to diagnose the cause of illness with no instrument other than his own hands, ears, eyes, and nose has perhaps been the aspect of acupuncture that has most impressed western doctors. There are a number of eminent American doctors who feel that the most up-to-date equipment and techniques are unable to reveal as much to them about a patient as is possible from an examination using the methods of acupuncture.

The Chinese doctor is trained to use four basic methods of diagnosis:

Asking: He finds out the background of the trouble, the symptoms, and so on.

Hearing: He is trained to listen to the sound of the voice as well as to what is said.

Seeing: He observes not only mechanical defects but also

the colors on certain parts of the face, the posture, and so on.

Feeling: He judges the texture of the skin, the variation in temperature of the skin surface, and finally he feels the Chinese pulses and thus finds the state of the vital energy flowing in the energy pathways to each of the respective organs and functions.

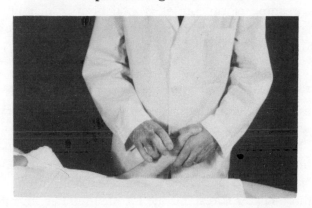

Other factors are also taken into account: the seasons, the moon phases, the time of day, smell, and the emotional or mental state of the patient. He will of course examine the patient thoroughly in the usual way.

All these methods direct him to the cause of the trouble, though the reading of the pulse is the most important.

In what sense is the pulse important in the acupuncturist's diagnosis? I thought the pulse could only reveal something about the heart and circulation.

The doctor of acupuncture is able to feel twelve different pulses on the wrists. He feels six on the left wrist, namely, the pulses of the heart, the small intestines, the liver, the gall bladder, the kidneys, and the bladder; and six on the right wrist, those of the lungs, the colon, the spleen, the stomach, "circulation-sex," and "three-heater." To many people brought up with the western ideas of pulse-taking, this seems very hard to believe. These twelve pulses are located at specific positions on the wrists and each one tells the exact state of the different organs or functions, and of the quantity and quality of the Ch'i energy passing through them.

The reading of the pulses is vital both to diagnosing the cause of disease and also to assessing the progress of the treatment.

What is meant by "circulation-sex" and "three-heater"?

These are both functions. Circulation-sex controls the arterial and venous blood and the internal and external sexual secretions. This particular function also has a very important role to play in mental disorders, as it is responsible for personal relationships, warmth, and affection among a host of other things. The three-heater is responsible for maintaining an even temperature in the upper, middle, and lower divisions of the body and for the harmony of temperature between the three divisions. This function again has tremendous implications in mental as well as physical disorders.

Why does the practitioner take into account the seasons, the moon phases, the time of day, and the emotional and mental state of the patient?

The Ch'i energy, the life force, is moving through the whole of creation and running through all life on this earth. Any alteration in the Ch'i energy of our environment will cause a reaction in the Ch'i energy in our bodies. There is a constant interplay between the two. Consider the rising of energy in the spring, the general increase of activity after the winter. Most people can feel this change within themselves.

All Ch'i energy is polarized, and is rather like the energy of a battery in that the positive side of the energy cannot exist on its own; the negative side of the energy must be there with it. The one cannot exist without the other. In the case of the Ch'i energy, however, the quality of the mixture is never constant. Sometimes one side becomes a little dominant, sometimes the other. During the day, for example, and at the time of the sun's rising in the sky, the active, positive side is a little dominant; during the night, the negative side of the energy (the rest and the dark) is a little dominant. But this dominance of one side or the other will also be affected by the phases of the moon, by the season of the year, by the weather, by the actual time of the day or night, and so on.

The balance of the Ch'i energy in a person's body will be further affected by his emotions, by his physical state—e.g., exhaustion—and by his mental state. He may be worried, depressed, and so on. He may be suffering from an inferiority complex, or from some hereditary factor.

All of these things will affect the Ch'i energy and the practitioner must take them all into consideration when reading the pulses.

The reading of the pulses is made more complicated by the fact that the total energy in the body is not distributed equally between the twelve main organs and functions. First one is dominant, then another, so that both the quantity of Ch'i energy in the particular meridian and its quality or balance between the positive and negative sides will be changing from time to time. It is only when due consideration has been given to these points that the practitioner will know whether the particular pulse is imbalanced and requires correction. Actually, imbalance becomes apparent in a pulse long before an illness is manifest in the body.

Why does the acupuncturist take into account colors and smells?

When a person is not in perfect health, his body smell, the color of his skin, and the sound of his voice are affected. There are certain distinctive signs in each of these three that act as pointers to the organ or function that is out of order. The signs are of course usually very slight, and long experience is needed to be able to read them. An experienced practitioner will, for instance, recognize the smell of fever as soon as he enters the patient's room. He will look for the color change especially on certain areas of the face.

All these signs are of particular use in corroborating what has been learned from reading the pulses.

Would the doctor of acupuncture be able to tell simply from these methods what, for example, was causing migraine?

Yes. The examination is the most crucial part of the whole system and the experienced practitioner can indeed determine the exact cause of sickness.

There are a multiplicity of reasons why a person may be suffering from migraine. It could be due to malfunctioning of the liver and/or the gall bladder, the malfunctioning of the stomach, the spleen, the kidneys, the colon, or the small intestines, and so on, or it might be of mental origin. It will only be by using the Chinese methods of diagnosis that the practitioner will know which of these organs is in disorder and causing the distress signal called migraine. It is only at this point that he is in a position to go ahead and treat the cause. As soon as this has been corrected, the symptom, the migraine, will disappear.

7.

The Consultation and Diagnosis before Starting Treatment

If I were going to a practitioner for the first time, should I expect the Chinese method of examination? And would this take a long time?

The first session will be a consultation and examination lasting about one and one half to two hours. The practitioner will ask about the present symptoms, the history of the trouble, and the nature of any pain, and may want to know something of the patient's life and family history. He may ask certain things about the patient that seem, on first hearing, to have little to do with the complaint, but it must be remembered that the doctor of acupuncture is viewing his patient as a whole person, body +mind together, and any aspect of his life may prove important in understanding the cause of the imbalance in his health.

The practitioner will then spend some considerable time examining the patient and reading the pulses. The examination is very thorough, the significance of physiology being perhaps somewhat deeper in nature in traditional Chinese medicine than it is in present western medicine. The findings from reading the twelve pulses will be perhaps the most important pointers to the cause of the trouble. All of the findings from the examination are subsequently considered and worked over in planning the treatment.

Does this mean that the practitioner will not be able to go straight on from the examination and give the first treatment?

Yes. Following the consultation the practitioner may need to spend some two to four hours working on the case notes and plan before he is ready to start treatment.

What sort of a diagnosis is given after the examination?

The patient should not expect a diagnosis in normal Western terms. After the consultation and the preliminary work on the case notes, one can expect to be told the causative factors of the illness and whether or not it is likely to respond to treatment.

It is our custom in the West to expect a name to be given to our illness, but this will not be done; no label will be attached to it. These named illnesses are, after all, only the manifestation of disease in the body. As *dis-ease* progresses in a body, causing ever more damage, the relatively minor symptoms with names such as gastritis and backache may develop into major symptoms of disorder with a new set of names such as stomach ulcers and arthritis.

If the cause is treated the symptoms will disappear of themselves. Take the case of a headache. Aspirin will allow temporary relief of the condition, but the real trouble is the causative factor, and this must be dealt with in order to remove the headache completely.

8.

The Treatment: Duration, Effects, Cost

How many treatments are usually necessary?

This varies considerably from person to person and one cannot be guided by the experience of other patients. Some patients may need less than eight treatments, others as many as eighty. A lot depends on the severity of the disease, how long the patient has suffered from it, what drugs have been or are being taken, and so on.

One hears of the occasional "miracle cure" by acupuncture when a chronic condition of very long standing has responded to acupuncture so rapidly that the patient is well after only half a dozen treatments, but this is very, very rare indeed. When an illness has become really deeply seated it is only to be expected that it will take a long time to rectify the trouble, and much patient work will be needed.

How frequent are the treatments?

This also varies, but on the average treatments are given twice a week for three weeks and then once a week. As the patient improves, visits will be reduced to once every two weeks and then once a month.

Will the benefits from the treatments be lasting, or must there be a follow-up course after a few months, or after a year or so?

This rests largely with the patient. Follow-up treatments should not be necessary if the patient is living sensibly, with moderate diet and habits, and is able to avoid undue stresses and strains.

But if the patient returns to the same conditions that caused the original trouble, of course it will happen again and more treatments will be necessary.

It would probably be sensible for the patient to come once a year for a check-up as the practitioner will be able to tell from the pulses if anything is going wrong in the body long before it manifests itself in some visible symptom. The average person doesn't wait until something has gone wrong before taking his car in to be checked. We should not pay less attention to our body!

What does the treatment and the initial consultation cost?

It is extremely difficult to give an indication of cost, as this of course will vary from practitioner to practitioner. The charges will be roughly in line with those of other medical practitioners.

Do doctors of acupuncture employ nurses as do western doctors?

Yes, they employ nurses.

How long does it take to give a treatment?

The average treatment takes about half an hour. The pulses are read and the needles put in position. These are left in position until the desired effect is achieved. This may take just a second or two, a few minutes, half an hour, or in some cases even longer. The response to the treatment is again checked and assessed from the pulses. The patient will usually be left to rest for twenty minutes or so while the needles are doing their work. During this resting time it is unusual for the patient even to feel where the needles are in the body.

Does the patient lie down or sit up for treatment?

Where possible the patient lies down, but he can be treated sitting up if for any reason it is necessary.

Are patients usually nervous about the treatment?

Yes, I think most patients are nervous. In fact I am sure that nine out of ten people have the impression that the insertion of a needle will be as painful as a hypodermic injection. After the examination I am only too happy to show a patient a needle and to demonstrate how it is inserted, usually just below the skin, so that he may come to his first treatment feeling more confident and relaxed. Once a patient has had his first treatment, he usually feels perfectly happy about further treatments.

Does the acupuncture practitioner encourage the patient to watch the needles go in?

It is really up to the patient whether or not he watches the needles inserted. Some patients prefer to lie back, close their eyes, and leave everything in the hands of the practitioner. Others watch eagerly each insertion and manipulation, and are anxious to know what every needle is doing.

Of these two attitudes perhaps the latter is more helpful to the patient as over his period of treatment he will learn more about his sickness and its cause and effect, and will probably gain a better understanding of how his body+mind functions.

How quickly can the patient hope to feel improvement?

This varies a good deal depending on the disorder, but a patient can usually expect to feel some benefit within four or five treatments.

Should the patient expect any reaction to the treatment? Would he feel worse before feeling better?

On the whole the discomforts caused are mild and will not prevent the patient from leading his normal life.

There may be an aggravation (or worsening) of the symptoms, but this will not last for long and the patient is usually told whether to expect any such reaction at the time of the first treatment. This aggravation can be taken as an encouraging sign as it shows that the condition is responding to the treatment and may be helped or cured. One of the laws of natural medicine states that disease must go from within outwards, from above to below, and that the symptoms will return in the reverse order from which they came, if one is to effect a cure. An aggravation can be seen as a "healing crisis" and the start of this outward movement on the part of the disease.

Usually an aggravation brings only slight discomfort to the patient, but in certain cases of deeply seated disease it can be quite severe. It will, however, last only for a short time, from perhaps an hour to a day. The practitioner clearly tries to avoid causing too severe a reaction but in certain cases he has no choice.

As someone who had been seriously ill for six years said to me the other day, "The important question is, can you get me better? I shouldn't mind about any temporary discomfort if I know that I am getting well."

Might one experience any other effects besides these aggravations?

The patient may feel very tired and sleepy after the first few treatments and may be advised to go home and have a rest for an hour or so.

The treatment may also result in looseness of the bowels, a cold, skin irritation or spots, sweating and so on—all signs that the body is responding and with the help of the treatment is ridding itself of poisons.

The reaction will depend largely on the organ or function of the body that is being treated. If, for example, a patient were suffering a lot of pain and heavy bleeding during menstruation, and the spleen was being treated to correct this, she might be surprised to find that she had a sudden desire for sweet things instead of the spicy foods she had always preferred, or, vice versa, a sudden desire for spicy foods and no inclination for the sweet things she had always been tempted to eat. (This is only temporary, and a balance will be reached as soon as the organ is functioning correctly.)

The practitioner's aim is gradually to balance the whole body + mind. All of these reactions resulting from treatment are caused by the regulation of the flow of vital energy through the body and the resultant reawakening of certain organs and functions that have been sluggish and the slowing down of the overactive ones."

Some people say that acupuncture can cause harmful side-effects. Is this true?

No. The patient would only have the type of reaction that we have been talking about, which would indicate that the disease was responding to treatment. I am, of course, talking about treatment given by a fully qualified practitioner.

Would the patient have to stop taking any drugs or medicine previously prescribed by other doctors?

Definitely not. It is most important that patients should tell their practitioner of any drugs or medicine that they are taking, but he will decide when the time is right for them to be slowly withdrawn. If a patient stops taking them immediately, he may suffer from withdrawal symptoms that will only worsen his general condition.

A patient should not take anything while undergoing treatment without first consulting his practitioner. Even such a simple medicine as an aspirin or indigestion tablet can interfere with the acupuncture treatment.

Does acupuncture do away with the need for internal medicines?

No. It may be necessary to give some form of internal medication along with the acupuncture treatment but this will be prescribed by the acupuncture practitioner and will be part of his whole plan for treating this disorder. This would usually be a natural medicine as prescribed in western herbalism and homoeopathy.

Is there any age limit for receiving treatment? Is acupuncture safe for children? And does it take longer for an older patient to get better?

There is no age limit, though a practitioner would not usually treat a child under seven years of age unless he were specially experienced. How long it takes to get better depends upon how long the patient has had the trouble rather than on his age. A person of seventy with a disease of a year's duration should get well faster than a person of thirty with a complaint of ten years' duration.

Can acupuncture do any harm when practiced by a fully qualified and competent practitioner?

No, none at all. The important thing is to make sure that the practitioner is indeed fully qualified.

9.

Rules to Observe before and after Treatment

Are there any instructions one should follow when receiving treatment?

Yes. Here are some things to do and not to do.

a. Do not bathe on the day of treatment. A light shower is permissible a couple of hours before or after.

b. Do not arrive rushed or hurried for treatment.

c. Do not eat a heavy meal before treatment or for 2 hours afterward.

d. After treatment, take things quietly for an hour or two.

Is there any way in which one can help the treatment to progress satisfactorily?

A sensible diet and moderate habits will certainly aid recovery and help keep a person in good health.

It is difficult today not to eat a lot of highly artificial foods with many additives and preservatives. This sort of food does not help the body to fight against disease as do more natural foods. The Ch'i energy running through the body, the life force, can be looked on as the gasoline on which our machine (our body) runs. Its tanks must constantly be refilled and the quality of the gas put into them will make all the difference to the smooth running of the motor. Our refueling is done from the air we breathe and the food we eat. And so the quality of the air and food put into the body is of great importance and will aid or impede its correct functioning.

It would be advisable to make the following simple changes in diet if the patient is eating the more artificial foods:

a. Replace white sugar and white sugar products with brown sugar and honey. (Note: It is not advisable to eat more than about four tablespoons of honey a day.)

b. Replace white flour and white flour products with whole meal products, preferably compost grown.

c. Increase salad intake.

d. Cook vegetables only lightly, keeping all possible nourishment.

e. Use condiments, sauces, and pickles sparingly if you cannot cut them out altogether.

f. Do not use canned foods.

g. Do not use foods preserved by chemicals or unnaturally prepared in any way.

One should aim to be moderate in all one's living habits.

10.

Differences in the Approach to Medicine between the West and Traditional East

Why hasn't the medical profession taken more interest in acupuncture and used it to treat disease along with more conventional methods?

It is not really surprising that acupuncture has not been readily accepted in the West because the two approaches to healing are very different. The two systems of medicine have developed from entirely different cultures and different needs. There are even observable differences between the general health of the West and of the East. Except in the large cities of China, which have adopted a western way of life, there is far less ill health generally, far less cancer, cardiac disease, and high blood pressure, and far fewer stress illnesses and mental disturbances than occur in the United States and similar countries.

The two medical systems tackle ill health from opposite ends of the whole problem. The western doctor has been trained to treat not the body + mind as a whole but a particular disorder. To do this he has various methods at his disposal. He may prescribe drugs to kill infection, to ease pain, to suppress and check a trouble, to supply a deficiency. He may operate to remove a diseased part of the body or to repair a part that has broken down. And so on. The traditional Chinese doctor looks upon all complaints as symptoms of trouble in the body, as manifestations of disease. He is trained to treat the cause, not the disorder, and tries to restore the life force to the parts of the body in which it was deficient so that the whole body is brought once again into balance. The disorder will then disappear of itself.

Then there is the question of proof. The western mind expects to have proof of the existence of something before it will believe in it. This is part of our whole upbringing. We prove in the classroom that metal expands when heated by seeing it with our eyes, and only then do we accept the fact.

It is understandable that the western doctor has found it difficult to believe in the existence of the meridians (energy pathways) and the acupuncture points (the points lying along the meridians that are used to control the energy), since they have not been found or recognized in the body in the course of dissection. Not until very recently has any trace of the Ch'i energy and its pathways appeared in any conventional scientific experiment. As the whole of the acupuncture treatment is based on controlling this Ch'i energy from the energy pathways, this is no small stumbling block. The fact that a sick person is brought back to full health by acupuncture does not and cannot stand as proof to the western scientist's mind that the principles upon which the Chinese have founded their medicine are valid. On the whole, the western doctor has been inclined to believe that the success of acupuncture must be due to the power of suggestion, faith in the healer, the fact of the illness being psychosomatic, and so on. This attitude is now changing somewhat, mainly as the result of Soviet and Korean research.

It is rather interesting that before 1960 the Russians led a medical research team in an attempt to disprove acupuncture and ended up so impressed with it that arrangements were made for training and research at six universities.

Despite the difficulty of belief in the meridian theory, etc., many doctors in the West have been so impressed by the acupuncturist's ability to diagnose, and very often to help, when conventional medicine has failed that they now show great interest in acupuncture. This is particularly so in the United States where many doctors are anxious to study the philosophy and principles of acupuncture, even though they may be unable to spend the necessary time to qualify as a practitioner. Large numbers of American doctors are also anxious to learn the Chinese techniques of diagnosis.

Is it because acupuncture is not yet fully accepted in the West that it isn't tried by most people until conventional medicine has failed?

Yes, this is probably the case. Despite this, there is still a very high rate of success. There are many case histories of sufferers from chronic arthritis, chronic asthma, diabetes, heart and circulatory disorders, migraine, and other so-called incurable diseases who have been fully restored to health by acupuncture. In some cases disease may have gone too far to bring about a complete return to health, but still much may be done to alleviate the condition. The job of the acupuncture practitioner would be so very much easier if he were able to treat these conditions before they become firmly rooted in the body.

11.

Acupuncture in China Today

Do the Chinese themselves still use acupuncture or have they adopted the conventional methods of medicine?

Western medicine was gradually introduced into China in about 1840, and by 1920 an attempt was even made to abolish traditional medicine. The Chinese Communist party, however, has been anxious for the western and traditional Chinese schools of medicine to cooperate with one another. Mao Tse-tung believes that traditional Chinese medicine is a great treasure house to be fully explored, and that anything of value should be used and improved wherever possible. Many Western-trained Chinese doctors have found it as difficult as our own doctors to accept and use these ancient arts; nevertheless, the Chinese medical world has now undergone a great change. Acupuncture and traditional Chinese medicines are used alongside Western methods in all branches of healing.

Research and reassessment of the traditional medicines is still in its early stages, but much good work has been done. Among recent developments, two particular instances have been frequently reported in the West: the healing of deaf-mute children; and the use of acupuncture for anesthesia.

Have the Chinese actually succeeded in completely curing deaf-mute children?

Yes. During the past four years work has been done on this problem and it is reported that many deaf-mutes have received their hearing and speech.

In 1968 a medical team of acupuncturists was sent to a school for deaf-mutes in Liaoyuan, in the Kirin province. The children there had been termed incurable. Acupuncture texts instruct that certain acupoints provide a stimulus for hearing and speech, but there were no recent accounts of deaf-mute people being cured. The team performed many experiments on themselves before beginning treatment on the children. As a result of this work they had great success in bringing back the hearing of these children, but not the speech at first.

One of the young Chinese doctors felt that the only way to stimulate the acupoint controlling speech sufficiently was to insert the needle to a greater depth, but all the people and reference material he could consult advised against this. It was believed that there was a danger that a normal person's speech would be impaired if the needle were inserted beyond a certain depth or even that his life would be endangered. This doctor decided to go ahead and experiment on himself. His belief proved correct. He found that full stimulation was not reached until the needle was inserted farther.

After more experiments on themselves the team worked for some considerable time to help the children. It is said that 157 of the school's 168 pupils regained their hearing, and 149 were able to speak. Since this time this treatment has been widely used throughout China and is still being improved.

This news appears to have been treated with skepticism if not ridicule by some doctors in the West. Surely it would be better to learn and try these new methods for ourselves rather than to condemn them untried. Imagine what it means to a person to receive his hearing and speech. As the young Chinese doctor who risked his own life said, if we refuse to try out new methods, then we should call deaf-mutes not incurables but rather cases refused treatment.

How is acupuncture used as a means of inducing anesthesia?

As in the case of the deaf-mutes, doctors in China today have been researching the old methods, in this instance of pain-killing; and they have experimented to find ways of completely anesthetizing different parts of the body so that a person may undergo surgery.

This is done quite simply by placing a few needles into specific points of the body, very often only two or four, usually in the lower legs and feet or lower arms. These needles are stimulated by the anesthetist, each in turn, for some fifteen to twenty minutes before the operation, and then at intervals during the operation. Sometimes this is done by hand, at other times electricity is used (although of course there is no electric current passing into the body). This action stimulates the acupoints.

This method is proving very successful. The patients are conscious throughout the operation and appear to be completely calm and relaxed about it. Their blood pressure, breathing, and pulse remain normal. In many cases the patient can cooperate with the surgeon, for instance, in regulating his breathing. There is still sensation in the anesthetized area, but no pain is felt. When the incision is made the patient feels as if a pencil is being run across his skin, and he is aware that an organ is being moved or that a bone is being cut, but that is all.

This method of anesthesia is proving particularly valuable to the Chinese, for they have such vast rural areas that it is virtually impossible to get patients needing urgent operations to a hospital in time or to get the anesthesia equipment out to them. Using acupuncture anesthesia, operations can take place anywhere. Great numbers of lives have already been saved by using this method.

In the West acupuncture anesthesia would make it possible to operate on those whose age, heart condition, and so on would expose them to serious danger if conventional anesthetics were used. Acupuncture anesthesia is also much less expensive than conventional methods and it has the great merit that the patient suffers no after-effects from it. In an emergency an operation can be performed immediately as there are none of the usual food difficulties. The patient may eat at any time before, during, or after the operation. The recovery time is very much speeded up, and after minor operations patients frequently feel well enough to walk back to their beds.

A person may learn to use acupuncture anesthesia in a *relatively* short time. He does not need the full training of the traditional doctor because he will be using acupuncture for this one use only; he will not be attempting to remove the cause of illness by regulating the vital energy in a patient.

12.

Soviet and Korean Research Substantiating Acupuncture

What traces of the meridians and Ch'i energy have actually been found in experiments?

A considerable amount of research has been done in recent years both in the Soviet Union and in Korea that has produced a great deal of evidence proving, in western scientific terms, the validity of traditional Chinese ideas and beliefs.

It is worth describing these experiments and findings in some detail. You may find, as did the Soviet scientists, that it is easier to believe in the principles and workings of acupuncture once you have been shown some concrete, scientific evidence of this vital energy and its pathways through the body. So I will set out as simply as possible some of the main points that have arisen from these experiments, which confirm what the Chinese have been saying for thousands of years.

The USSR

The real breakthrough came in 1939 when two Soviet scientists, S. D. and V. Kirlian, discovered a method of observing and photographing living substance in high-frequency electrical fields. The results were remarkable. Some sort of energy was seen to be constantly moving through the living tissues that showed up as multicolored lights, sparks, flares, channels of light, and so on being discharged from the hand, say, or the leaf that was being observed under the lens of the microscope.

After thirteen years or so of experiments it was concluded that all living things, both plants and animals, have both a physical body and an energy body. Any imbalance seen in the energy body was in time reflected in the physical body. The Kirlians found that from examining this energy body they could foresee illness both in plants and in themselves. Further, this energy body had an existence of its own. A leaf with a third of it cut off, or a human body that was minus a limb, was seen to still have a complete energy body—a sort of ghost of the missing part was still there.

The energy pattern in the body was found to be affected very rapidly by emotions, states of mind, thoughts, alcohol and other things, as well as illness and pain. When a person was tired or very tense, far more energy was seen to pour out of the body, and at a much greater rate. The greater the pain in an area, the more brilliant were the lights given off from this area.

This energy body has been much spoken of by different religions and philosophies under such names as the subtle body, the astral body, the etheric body, and so on, and by acupuncturists as the vital energy or life force. But scientists on the whole have always held the existence of this subtle body much in question. Except for the fact that Dr. Walter J. Kilner of St. Thomas's Hospital, London, had discovered at the beginning of this century that the human aura became visible when a person was looked at through specially stained glass screens, this was really the first time that scientists had been able to fully see and study this second energy body of a living being, and they were amazed by what was revealed under Kirlian photography.

Much excitment was created among leading Soviet scientists from very many different fields.

It wasn't until 1953 that a Leningrad surgeon, Dr. M. K. Gaikin, realized that these Kirlian photographs and the subsequent experiments were giving visible proof to the premises of acupuncture. He had noticed that the position of the main flares on the skin did not correspond to the position of the nerve endings and could not be electrical energy. Also, these same flares were to be seen issuing from plants, and plants have no nervous system. It suddenly crossed his mind that these energy flares might be appearing on the identical spots that the Chinese had charted as their acupoints (the points from which the vital energy is manipulated). All of his subsequent research substantiated his hunch.

Assertions Made by Acupuncture
And the Soviet Findings Supporting These

Ch'i Energy

The acupuncturists talked for nearly five thousand years of the vital energy or life force. Here at last, in the twentieth century, the Kirlian photography made it visible to all.

Meridians and Acupoints

According to acupuncture, the energy flows along specific pathways or meridians connecting the organs deep in the body with the acupoints on the surface of the body.

The Russian experiments showed that this energy does indeed take interior pathways and does not travel along the surface of the body. The channels of light leading to the surface of the body that showed up under the Kirlian photography did seem to tie up with the Chinese chartings of the meridians or energy pathways, and the flares did indeed seem to issue from the acupoints.

Positive and Negative Yang and Yin

The traditional Chinese conception is that this vital energy is polarized into the positive and negative Yang and Yin, and that this is quite separate from the electrical energy in a body.

Scientists at the Kirov State University of Kazakhstan found that this newly visible body was indeed polarized but not electrical. (The Kirlians noticed that the light flares seen coming from the body seemed to be of two basic colors, blue and a reddish-yellow.)

Interplay between body+mind and the cosmos

The Chinese have always said that there is a constant interplay between the mind, the body, and the environment—all linked by the vital energy—and that the positive and negative aspects of the one vital energy are constantly fluctuating as they are affected by the continuous shift of things: by changes in the universe, by weather, seasons, moon phases, and so on; by moods, emotions, thoughts; by mental disturbances and physical illness.

The findings by the group of researchers at Kazakhstan all agreed with these assertions. This bioplasmic body, as they called the energy body, was seen to be affected by the atmosphere and by all cosmic occurrences. Disturbances of the sun, for example, change the whole plasmic balance of the universe, resulting in measurable physical changes in organisms. The Kirlians had already noticed the very rapid and marked effects of strong emotions and moods on the energy body, the increased light pouring out with anger and exhaustion, for example. And it was seen that emanations of thought and mood and emotion affect other living things as well as the physical body of the initiator.

When the hands of a "healer" were held close to a patient

under the Kirlian camera, the energy coming from the hands became concentrated into a small channel of intense light that beamed onto the area of illness. Healing in this instance seemed to show a transfer of energy from the bioplasmic body of the healer to that of the patient. Water that has been held in the hands of depressed psychiatric patients has been found to retard the growth of seeds whereas that held in the hands of a healer has increased growth.

All of these observations led the Soviet scientists to believe that man is indeed very much more closely linked to and affected by all life and the cosmos than they had previously thought possible.

The highest form of medicine is preventive medicine

Acupuncture is based on the principle that the highest healing science works with the invisible Ch'i energy and not with the physical body, and that a master of acupuncture is able to prevent disease in the physical body by noting and correcting any imbalance that appears in this vital energy.

One of the things that most impressed the Kirlians was that they could foresee disease in an organism, and Soviet scientists quickly realized the importance of such information. They saw that a knowledge of acupuncture would help them to interpret these changes in the energy pattern—changes in color, in intensity of light, and so on—and lead them to diagnose the type of illness that would appear in the physical body if the energy body were not restored to its normal state.

Each individual is unique

Acupuncture has always believed that the whole of each individual is unique, the pattern of his vital energy as well as his mind and physical body. Consequently no two patients can ever be treated alike; each must be viewed as a whole and separate organism, body+mind together, joined by the vital energy in a unique relationship with the whole creation.

The Kazakhstan scientists stated that this second energy body "is not just particles. It is not a chaotic system. It is a whole unified organism in itself," having shape, and being quite specific for each different organism. (Just as an oak leaf is recognizable as an oak leaf and no other leaf, so too is the energy body of an oak leaf recognizable as the energy body of an oak leaf and of no other leaf.)

Renewing the Ch'i Energy

The Chinese say that the Ch'i energy in a person is replenished from the air we breathe and the food we eat. According to the Kazakhstan scientists, some of the electrons and a certain amount of the energy in the oxygen we breathe are taken into the energy body. They were able to watch this process as it was happening. Breathing, they say, renews the vital energy and helps to restore any imbalance in the energy body.

Despite the large amount of information that was collected about this bioluminescence by the Kirlian camera, it was not until 1968 that the scientists at the Kirov State University of Kazakhstan in Alma-Ata finally made their statement that all living things, both plants and animals, have both a physical body of atoms and molecules and a counterpart energy body. They called this the biological plasma body, plasma being a fourth state of matter, masses of ionized particles—electrons, protons, and possibly others.

This confirmation by leading Soviet scientists of the suppositions made from the Kirlian findings can really be regarded as a landmark in the progress of western scientific understanding, for it is of major significance in practically all fields of science. Among other things it opens the gate to a whole group of subjects that have always been viewed with suspicion by the western scientific mind, such things as telepathy, extrasensory perception, and psychic healing. One of the sciences to receive its western seal of approval is acupuncture. It has now been fully accepted in the USSR; it is used alongside conventional western medicine and is studied in many of the top Soviet medical institutes.*

Korea

The work that Professor Kim Bong Han and his team of scientists are doing in Korea substantiates the existence of meridians and acupoints and shows how the flow of the life force in the meridians affects the body+mind.

They find that there is an integrated system of ducts that form a network entirely independent of the vascular, lymphatic, blood, and nervous systems. They call this the Kyungrak system. It is made up of four sets of ducts, all of them linked by terminal ductules much as the arteries and veins are linked by tiny blood vessels. These ducts are the meridians of acupuncture.

Not only have the Korean researchers been able to locate the meridians, but they have also done very detailed investigations of the fluids contained in these ducts. The team has injected a radioisotope into an acupoint, and has been able to watch the flow of the meridian fluid from the acupuncture point on the skin inward to the deeper ducts, and then finally outward again. This has resulted in radiophotographic plates that actually reveal the paths of these meridians running through the body.

Experiments have been performed that show how an organ in the body is controlled by a particular meridian. The meridian has been severed and the changes that take place in the organ observed.

*Much of what is given here about Soviet research is from Sheila Ostrander and Lynn Schroeder, *Psychic Discoveries Behind the Iron Curtain* (New York: Bantam Books, 1971).

Fig. 1. Model of Superficial Bonghan corpuscle

1.) Hair
2.) Epidermis
3.) Radiating smooth muscle fibre
4.) Outer layer
5.) Inner substance
6.) Superficial Bonghan duct
7.) Profund Bonghan duct
8.) Skeletal muscle

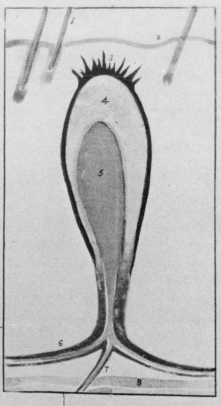

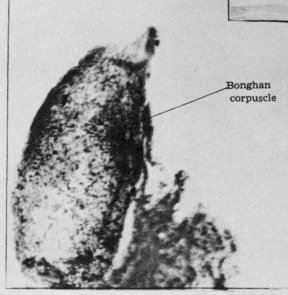

Bonghan
corpuscle

Fig. 2. Superficial Bonghan
corpuscle (16×16)

The team has found that there is a very important constituent of the meridian fluid, which they have named Sanal. It is a unique type of granule and contains DNA, RNA, and protein. It is involved in the formation of cells: Sanal, identified by a radioisotope, fuses into a cell from the meridian fluid, and later breaks down and recirculates as Sanal; apparently at a certain stage it becomes indistinguishable from the chromosomes of the cell. Kim Bong Han feels that the hereditary factors attributed to the chromosomes are in fact part of the work of Sanal. He has also found that the type of cell formed is dependent on whether the Sanal granules are taken from one meridian or another: this is to say that a liver cell can only be formed from Sanal that flows in the meridian that controls the liver. This network of meridians is one of the first things to form in an embryo (within fifteen hours of conception in a chick) and is thought to play an important part in the formation of the different organs as the body grows.

All of Professor Kim Bong Han's work, although extremely complex and detailed, can be looked at very simply. He is explaining in biochemical terms exactly how it is that the Kyungrak system of ducts—the acupuncturist's network of meridians —plays so vital a part in the smooth functioning of the organs of the body, and consequently affects the condition of the whole physical body. The practitioner of acupuncture is going straight to a controlling power when he treats a patient through this network of meridians in the body.*

The kind of experiments that the Soviets and Koreans have been carrying out appeals strongly to the western mind. Their scientific approach persuades us of the truth of their findings. And this is good. Knowledge must always be expressed in the

*For further reading see Academy of Medical Sciences, *Journal of D.P.R.K.* (Pyongyang, Korea: Medical Science Press, 1965).

life-style and language of each different culture for it to be accepted and believed.

It must be remembered, however, that this knowledge is not new. It is being rediscovered for western technological civilization. The truths that are reappearing in the West have always been the foundations of acupuncture, the traditional Chinese system of medicine. The system is founded on a true understanding of man and his relationship to the cosmos, and this fact is enabling it to live on after the death of the old Chinese civilization in which it grew up and to move into a completely new, materialistic, technological civilization.

13.

Acupuncture's Role in the Prevention of Disease

If the acupuncturist saw a patient early enough, could he prevent disease from developing?

Certainly. The doctor of acupuncture would be able to tell from the pulses if any "body function" was not in full working order a long time before any sort of disease could develop.

Would an acupuncture practitioner be willing to give a person a check-up from time to time to find out if there was anything starting to go wrong in the body?

Yes, he would. Perhaps the greatest contribution to health that acupuncture can make is as a preventive system of medicine. In order to encourage this practice, many doctors of acupuncture would be willing to charge a smaller fee for a check-up.

It was because of the acupuncturists' ability to prevent illness that the Chinese used to keep or pay their doctor only when they were well. Indeed, if they became ill, the Mandarin classes frequently dispensed with the services of their doctor or beheaded him!

*Is it likely that the medical profession will swing farther
toward preventive medicine?*

Many eminent doctors and other people concerned with all
aspects of health and welfare are now saying that if we in the
West are to be able to cope with the ever-increasing demands
on all the health services, there must be a completely new
approach to tackling the problem. Our present system of health
care is inadequate. Already in the United States there are barely
enough doctors to go around; it is exceedingly difficult to get a
bed in a hospital when it is needed; and many thousands of
people, if too ill to get to the doctor themselves, simply have to
do without proper medical attention because so many doctors
are too busy to visit.

The number of people needing help for illness brought on
through the strains of modern living is soaring every year. Every day more and more people of all ages are turning to drugs
as an escape from their problems.

Dr. Kit Pedler, a Research Fellow at the Institute of Ophthal-
mology, London, who has had both clinical practice and long
research experience, said recently on British television that we
must begin by changing radically our methods of training doctors. The emphasis must be away from specialization and iso-
lated research and back to the old-fashioned relationship of the
family doctor. In Pedler's view, students should spend less time
in hospitals and more time studying with a doctor in practice
and out doing social work. The aim would be to finish with a
broader understanding of the overall problems of living and
health, and a greater sympathy and general understanding of
how people live in our society. A doctor's duty should lie in
keeping his own community healthy and happy. People must
visit their doctor regularly for a check-up, just as they do the
dentist, and not wait until they are ill. Each patient must be

treated as an individual and given sufficient time to help with all of his or her problems. The pressure of numbers must be taken off our present general practitioners by directing a much greater proportion of qualified men and women into general practice; and far more attention must be paid to educating people in all matters of health from school age on.

If in the coming years this changed attitude became generally accepted, with the emphasis on keeping people well rather than on curing them once ill, then the philosophies underlying the two systems of medicine, those of the West and of the traditional East, would certainly draw much closer together. Dr. Pedler's ideas are very much in line with traditional Chinese thinking.

The Chinese have always said that each person must be treated as an individual, with respect not only to his body and to his mind, but also to his unique relationship with his environment. The vital energy in each person has its own special harmony with the Ch'i energy of the universe. Although the Ch'i energy in every person is affected by the same influences—cosmic happenings, weather, moon phases, seasons, and so on—each person has his own unique balance, dependent on his own particular vital energy body.

Any moves on the part of western medicine to give doctors the time and opportunity to understand each patient as an individual in his own circumstances and environment must be beneficial. And so too must be any moves to teach people how to keep themselves healthy.

Prevention of disease is of the very greatest importance, and is something that the Chinese people once took so much as a matter of course that they considered their doctor a poor one indeed if he were not able to keep them well. The doctor of acupuncture can play a vital part in the prevention of ill health, as the Soviets have already realized. Warning signals are always present in our body+mind when it is getting out of balance, and the practitioner of acupuncture can detect this imbalance in the vital energy from reading the pulses and other indications; he can correct this imbalance before it has time to manifest itself as physical illness.

But it is all too easy for the patient to become ill again unless he has understood why the illness came about and has taken steps to prevent its recurrence.

The attitudes of western society will have to change if the medical profession is to have any success with campaigns to prevent disease. Society must become much more aware of the effect of our way of living on general health and must be willing to make and pay for certain changes in this life-style.

This is where there is such a big difference between the practice of acupuncture in the western world today and its practice in China centuries ago. Any form of medicine today is a battle to keep people well when the whole way of western life is driving them toward illness. In ancient China there was a much slower pace of living, and people grew up believing that all order, tranquillity, and happiness, and consequently health, stemmed from the effort of each individual to follow The Way (the Tao). This would be roughly similar, in western language, to seeking to serve God or Truth rather than seeking to serve oneself. Each man's primary work was to bring about a balance and harmony within himself and into his own life. Once this was achieved, this balance and harmony would spread out in ever-widening circles into the family and the home, into the small communities of village and town, and on to encircle the whole of the country. It would move into and influence all aspects of work from the immediate needs of the family and neighbors to the politics and government of the country and to the production of all necessities and works of art. In such a way of life general health was much better, and the task of the doctor of acupuncture to keep people well was much easier.

For the situation to improve here in the West each individual person will need to realize that he himself can do a great deal toward keeping himself healthy. People today all too readily go to their doctor expecting him to make them well once they are ill. How much better it would be if every person were able to work with his doctor, seeking his guidance on how to *keep* himself well.

If Western life is driving people toward illness, is there very much an individual can do to keep himself healthy?

Every individual can do a great deal about his health, although now it is not easy for any western person to lead the sort of natural existence that encourages health. The ideal would be to eat pure food, to drink pure water, breathe pure air, to work at a pace and time in harmony with natural laws, to be free from stresses, and generally to live in tranquillity and happiness in close union with nature, all creation, and God.

Each individual must first accept a good deal of responsibility for keeping himself well. Of course certain difficulties and stresses cannot be avoided; things will go wrong, accidents will happen, he will not notice his danger signals or he will choose to ignore them. Ill health will result and doctors and medical facilities will be needed. But there are countless cases of illness, physical and mental, that need never occur if people, from childhood, were given an understanding of their bodies and minds and their needs, and of the interrelationship of all life on earth, and the relationship of life on earth with the universe.

It may be helpful to know the factors to which the Chinese attribute ill health. First, a man may suffer mechanical or chemical injury. Second, a man may become diseased in body or mind. Disease, the Chinese believe, is caused by the interaction between the internal condition of a man and the external world, and there are certain internal and external factors that may bring about illness. Internally a man may be subjected to fear, grief, anger, worry and anxiety, joy, and may be affected by constitutional hereditary factors. Externally he may be subjected to environmental changes: cold, heat, dryness, humidity, damp, wind, and fire. We will all at certain times be exposed to every one of these internal and external factors, and a healthy body+mind will be able to cope with them. For example, we may be angry or worried, or be exposed to excessive heat or damp, but after a short time our bodies readjust and are none the worse for it. But when the body is subjected to a continued excess of any of the above factors, the Ch'i energy will be affected and will become imbalanced, thereby causing symptoms to appear internally or externally in the body+mind.

In the case of infectious and contagious diseases, the Chinese believe that if a person is in perfect health his body will resist infection. It is only the fact that our resistance has been lowered by one of the above factors that causes us to "catch" the illness.

As I have said, our way of life subjects us to a great many stresses and strains that can only lead to increasing breakdowns in the health of the body+mind. Collectively we are responsible for this present situation. It is our way of life. Certainly it has freed us from many of the dangers that faced our forefathers, and perhaps there is a lot of truth in the claim that the ordinary working man has never had such easy living conditions. But this technological age has created its own problems and difficulties, and it is only by understanding them and uniting in an attempt to right or better them that we will be able to create better conditions for our health.

The environment is of vital importance when considering the health of a people. The acupuncture practitioner cannot stand apart and heal people, as it were, in a vacuum. They have to be made well and kept well within their own society and way of life. In order to lessen the causative factors of illness it must be part of the duty of all concerned with healing to point out and urge out action wherever our way of living leads to ill health.

Much has already been written about our environment and Western way of life. This subject is so crucial to our health, however, that I am including as an appendix to this book a section showing just how we are affected by a high standard of living, a growing population, and the arms and space race. Even if much of the material is familiar to you, consider it this time purely from the standpoint of health.

But don't people live longer in our present society than ever before? And with the help of modern medicine aren't they kept free from many illnesses that had previously been regarded as fatal?

Yes, it is true that the life expectancy of man in the West has increased. This has been brought about both by better living accommodations, hygiene, and adequate food that is part of our high standard of living, and also by the skills and knowledge of modern medicine in preventing disease (particularly the contagious diseases and the diseases of malnutrition) and in surgery.

The fact remains that such things as cancer, cardiac disease, high blood pressure, diabetes and nephritis, nervous weaknesses and mental disturbances—such as anxieties, depressions, loneliness—and the general reliance upon drugs, tranquilizers, stimulants, sleeping pills, multivitamins, and the like are always increasing in the United States and other countries following a similar life-style. Great strides have certainly been made in certain branches of medicine, but this is no reason for us to fail to acknowledge and try to correct the new difficulties facing us in modern Western life.

In the last few years there has been a growing appreciation of ecological dangers, and much has already been done to deal with the threats to health arising from our society. Nevertheless, much more has to be done. People have tolerated so many of these harmful situations only because they have been ignorant of the consequences, have simply not believed in the dangers, or have been reckless in the pursuit of profit. In this respect, at least, the situation is more hopeful now.

Along with this growing understanding of ecological dangers, isn't there also a growing dissatisfaction with the mad chase of life?

It is encouraging that people are beginning to realize the fruitlessness of seeking happiness by the pursuit of material things and temporary pleasures. Over the past few years we have seen a whole rash of "groups" appearing on the scene, all searching for something to make their lives more meaningful and to bring them contentment and happiness. There has been a great surge of interest in the philosophies of the East—in Taoism, Zen, Hinduism, and Buddhism; in yoga and meditation; in Christianity, with new movements emerging such as the Jesus Movement; in spiritualism; in ESP, telepathy and psychic happenings; in diet—vegetarianism, macrobiotic eating, health and compost-grown natural foods, health cures; and in a host of other things.

Unconventional life-styles are being tried out in attempts to reconnect with the natural rhythms of life and to become an integrated and vital part of a community. Hence we see people establishing communes, camps, "houses," and groups of all sorts, each creating a new environment, a little island of self-rule with its own aims and disiplines.

Isn't there a similar dissatisfaction with the modern approach to medicine and science?

Yes. Over the last decades western medicine has made rapid advances in many directions and has acquired far greater skills in surgery and the transplant of organs; it has developed very much more complicated medical machinery and equipment, and has introduced countless new and more powerful drugs. Research has been of the first importance, and specialization on a large scale has resulted from the complexity of information discovered.

It is true that many medical practitioners as well as many of the general public now feel that in this medical world of advanced technology, research, and specialization, the individual patient is becoming of little significance. All the attention is directed to the ailment, while the importance of the patient as a whole human being in a particular set of circumstances is overlooked.

Consequently an increasing interest has been shown in so-called "fringe medicines" over the past few years—such treatments as chiropractic, osteopathy, herbalism, homoeopathy, spiritual healing, hypnosis, and, among all these, acupuncture. These different treatments are all able to give one vital thing to the patient—individual attention. This means that you and your difficulty are of importance.

There are signs that a move away from specialization is beginning in many areas of science. Some researchers are now saying that it is imperative that they get back into touch with the whole scheme of creation, know where their own studies fit in and what other people's work is about.

It is so often thought that science and technology now have the answers to almost any questions about the universe, that it is no longer necessary to surround any areas with myth and mystery. But, while many people have been persuaded toward atheism or agnosticism by scientific findings, the pendulum has started to swing the other way. One now hears the occasional scientist (particularly one working in cosmology) say that he has never before seen so clearly that he knows so little, and that we are barely scratching the surface of knowledge. Far from feeling atheistic, he now stands awed before the enormity of these mysteries.

Having looked at some of the ways in which our life in the West today encourages ill health and having decided that there is a growing dissatisfaction with our life-style, what are some ways for an individual to help himself to stay healthy?

Perhaps the most important thing of all is to get one's values straight. Those people who have become dissatisfied with the technological rat race and are seeking to find a richness and purpose in life have already taken the turn toward healthy living. They are searching for that which is true, just, and lovely. And where they find it is really of little importance: whether in a religion or philosophy, in art or music, in a new style of living that takes them closer to nature and natural law, in knowledge, in pure science, or simply in the seeking of satisfaction in the tasks of one's daily life and in simple pleasures. No matter where we start, the end is ultimately the same and the important thing is that we are all united in the desire to satisfy the whole of our nature and not only our physical bodies.

Once this has happened everything else will fall into place. Our attitude toward life and toward work and pleasure and possessions will quite naturally alter. We shall cease to place such importance on pleasures and possessions. We shall cease to work for what we can get out of it and begin to discover the enjoyment of seeing what we can put into it. We shall find more time to enjoy the things that are freely given to all men—the sky, the birds, the trees, the company of our fellow men. We shall see more and hear more, know what is calling for attention, what needs to be done. We will begin to find a richness in living that eluded us when we were caught up in the rush and bustle.

When our outlook has changed in this way we shall be moving toward a mental harmony that will automatically affect the state of our physical body. Our Ch'i energy will become stronger and better balanced, thus enabling our physical body to function correctly.

But there are still certain things that we need to do.

We all need to pay regular attention to caring for our bodies and minds. The body is such a wonderful piece of machinery that we are inclined to forget all about it until it goes wrong. If only we would care for our body as we do our car—feed it on the best fuel, clean it, rest it sufficiently, have it checked regularly, and not drive it at a suicidal rate. You have only to look into a doctor's office to see countless people who have waited until it is too late, until the damage has been done and the body's mechanism has broken down. Only then do they give it their attention. (This would never have happened to their car.)

In ancient China the emphasis was always on a simple way of life. The people sought both to live moderately and to cultivate a moderate temperament. They sought to eat and live simply and not to work too hard or to strive for excessive gains. They strove to commit no acts of excess, to control their thoughts and personal feelings and not to give expression to the emotions that rose up inside them, to be unperterbed by success or failure, and to refrain from worry, from ambition, and so on. The three great philosophies of China—Taoism, Buddhism, and Confucianism—all advocate in their different ways this doctrine of the Mean or moderate, and the cultivation of this calmness of the heart or emotions, and control of the mind.

This approach to life was very deeply rooted in Chinese culture and its wisdom can be seen from the beneficial effects it had upon the body+mind. Many Chinese lived to be a good age; one hundred years was considered by them the perfect life span for a man. They suffered little from many of the present diseases of the West. Few of them contracted the diseases resulting from excessive worry and stress—diseases of the cardiac organs, of the nervous system, disturbances of the mind, cancer, and tumors. Few of them suffered from diabetes and nephritis, the results of excessive labor. And few of them suffered from high blood pressure. Certainly their diet contained little animal fat.

If we can follow the Chinese example, live moderately and cultivate a moderate temperament, we shall go a long way toward avoiding ill health.

We can try to introduce this discipline of moderation into our feeling and our thinking—the calmness of heart and control of the mind of the Chinese. But it is not something that can be achieved overnight. We all know, for example, the power that worry and anxiety can have over us. They can very quickly make us feel ill, and we begin to work inefficiently. Our minds become dominated by these worrying thoughts. It is only by constantly turning to the needs of the moment and by giving full attention to what we are doing that we can stop the worry having a constant negative effect upon us and draining our strength. To learn to discipline the mind and the emotions in this way can occupy a man for his whole life. But it is worth the effort since the reward will be great. It leads to the health of the whole man, to the peace of mind and inner happiness that all people desire, as well as to the health of the body.

We can also try to introduce this discipline of moderation into our living habits. In doing this we shall be caring for our bodies. We must allocate the necessary time to work and to play, to exercise the body and to rest it (and this includes sleeping at night in harmony with the earth and the sun, and not trying to turn night into day). And we must make time each day to be alone, and to be quiet. In this time we may choose to pray, or to commune with nature, to meditate, to practice relaxation, or simply to sit quietly and let go of everything. Any of these will refresh us and pull us off the ever-moving treadmill of activity. We can become one with ourselves again.

We can do our best to eat at regular times and in moderation, and to see that our diet is wholesome and balanced. Such a diet would consist as far as possible of fresh food (not frozen, canned, or preserved), that is uncontaminated by sprays, and food that is natural (not prepared unnaturally, and not containing additives).

We need to eat plenty of compost-grown whole cereals and grains (from which nutrients such as wheat germ have not been removed). We can do so either as whole-meal bread and whole-meal flour products, or as buckwheat, unpolished rice, whole wheat, barley and rye, crushed oats, etc. The legumes and certain seeds are very nutritious and a valuable source of protein. If we supplement our diet with these—such as split peas and beans, soya beans, lentils, nuts, sesame and sunflower seeds, Chinese sprouting beans—it isn't necessary to eat too much meat and cheese, both of which eaten in excess will put too much animal fat into the body. Plenty of vegetables, salad, and fruits should be eaten, preferably those that are fresh and in season. To sweeten food we should use brown sugar and honey.

No food should be eaten in excess. In the West we are very inclined to eat too much sweet and rich food and not enough fresh fruit and vegetables. It is important that we do not overload our bodies with sugar—cakes and puddings, candies, soft drinks, cookies. Nor should we eat much rich fatty food—such as cakes and puddings again, large quantities of butter on bread and in cooking, cooked foods using drippings and lard, fried foods (particularly French fried potatoes), cream, excessive milk and cheese, sherry, port and vermouth, chocolate.

The final point is that we should drink our food and eat our drinks. This is to say that we should chew our food thoroughly until it becomes liquid in the mouth, and that we should drink liquids slowly, a little at a time, holding it in the mouth long enough for it to be mixed with saliva. The way we eat is even more important than what we eat. It is of great importance that the process of digestion and assimilation should be started correctly, and this cannot happen unless all food and liquid is adequately mixed with saliva in the mouth.

We must not become slaves to our habits. The occasional cigarette or cigar and the occasional alcoholic drink, perhaps at the odd social gathering, will do us no harm. After a heavy day some people may find that it helps them to relax, and think of it as a means of releasing tension. The important thing to remember again is moderation. All too often, if we do not keep a strict watch upon ourselves, the occasional this or that can lead to excess, and we find we are subjecting our bodies to a new stress. This applies to all the things we do. Too many late nights, too many parties, too much entertaining, too many evening activities, too much television, too much physical work or exercise, too much mental work, too much talking, too much eating, too much sleeping—any of these things can lead to ill health.

Each one of us is different and what is right for one is wrong for another. Each of us must try to discover the needs and requirements of his own body+mind, and then use his common sense to keep within his limitations. It is not necessary to become fanatical and to go through life worrying about whether we should do this or that. The body is a remarkable organism and will be able to cope with most things if done occasionally, but it cannot be expected to stand up to continuous strain.

Finally, we can all take the time and trouble to teach our children from a very early age to strive for a healthy body+ mind and to learn the importance of moderation. To indulge a child with anything in his formative years is to guide him into habits that can only be injurious to his health. Children should learn about the wonders of the mechanism of the body, and its closely linked relationship with the mind and with the whole of creation. They should learn that the great riches of life are those that are freely given to men, and that the opportunity is theirs to enjoy these God-given things on earth. If they follow the right way, the doctrine of the Mean or moderation, their lives should be both long and rich. They have the potential for being happy and healthy in almost any situation if they have a true sense of values and understand that their happiness is not dependent on position, wealth, and material things; and that a life cannot be measured in years but in the richness of each moment.

Thus we have seen that there are three ways in which acupuncture can make a positive contribution to the prevention of ill health: (1) *by traditional diagnosis*—by feeling imbalance in the energy body and thus foreseeing disease before it is manifested in the physical body; (2) *by treatment*—by correcting the imbalance in the energy body before it has time to create disease in the physical body; (3) *by teaching*—by supplying a guideline to our living that will bring about improved health. In this last category, I hope to have shown that the ancient Chinese teachings are as applicable today as they ever were.

Do you see this guidance on healthy living as part of the work of the doctor of acupuncture today? Is his time not fully occupied in trying to restore the sick to health?

This is certainly a problem for the present-day practitioner. Very often, much as he would like to help and guide people who are at present well and who seek his advice in "check-ups," for the most part he feels that the seriously sick person who has turned to him for help must take priority. It is perhaps only in small ways, such as helping to spread the information in this chapter, that the present-day doctor of acupuncture is able to carry out his duty to improve general health by encouraging and urging a moderate way of life.

The aim to act as a counselor and thus to improve general health was always a very important one to the true servant of acupuncture. The approach to medicine in ancient China was very broad. This can perhaps be seen best by turning briefly to a part of the *Nei Ching,* the book that remains the foundation of acupuncture. The Yellow Emperor was talking to his First Minister, Ch'i Po, and seeking instruction on all questions of health and the art of healing. He urged Ch'i Po to tell him about Nature, Heaven, and Tao (the Way), and asked to be informed about their workings. He wished to understand the workings of Nature to the utmost degree, including full information about man, his physical form, his blood, his breath of life, his flowing, and his dissolution. He wanted to know what causes his death and his life. And he wished for advice on what can be done about all these things.

This gives us just a glimpse of the Chinese approach to medicine. It did not exist on its own and could not be studied on its own as a separate science. It was very closely tied up with man's understanding of life itself and of all creation. The art of healing was part of philosophy and religion, both of which advocated oneness with nature and the universe; and the man of medicine had to study and understand the ancient Chinese philosophy containing the three basic ideas common to all Chinese culture —the Tao, Yang and Yin, and the five elements. He had to concern himself with all such matters, as well as with anatomy and physiology, if he were to gain wisdom and understanding in his science.

The early master of acupuncture was therefore much more than merely his patients' medical man. He concerned himself with their full welfare and was their guide and instructor, helping them to follow a way of life that would keep their bodies, minds, and spirits at all times in close harmony with natural law and with the whole of creation.

Even today, in spite of the difficulties of the modern world, the doctor of acupuncture must keep these same aims in mind, both to prevent disease and, where it has occurred, to prevent a repetition.

14.

The Training and Qualifications of a Practitioner and a Warning against Unqualified Practitioners

How long must one train to become proficient in the art of acupuncture?

The Chinese consider that it takes up to ten years to become technically competent and much longer to become a master of acupuncture. The ability to read the pulses is the most difficult skill to acquire, and many years' experience of pulse-taking is needed to differentiate accurately between the twelve pulses and between the different qualities of each pulse. (The Chinese texts state that there are twenty-seven different qualities of each pulse.)

No better treatment can be found than good acupuncture, but bad acupuncture can be dangerous. It is quite wrong to think that even if it cannot do good, simply to stick a few needles under the skin cannot do any harm. Such an idea is terribly wrong. Acupuncture treatment is capable of doing great good, but if wrongly applied it can do great harm.

Where should a person go for treatment? And how would he know if the practitioner offering treatment were a qualified one?

There are unfortunately, as yet, only relatively few fully qualified practitioners in the West and less at the present time in the United States than in Great Britain and Europe. This is largely due to the difficulty of obtaining a complete training by traditional Chinese methods.

The College of Chinese Acupuncture (U.K.) was opened in England in 1961 to train Westerners strictly by traditional methods and up to the standards required by the Chinese colleges. Since then, many people have passed the college's examinations and are now qualified and registered practitioners. Most of these people are practicing in England, though some have scattered throughout the world. No student of this college may practice on his own until he holds the qualification Licentiate of Acupuncture (Lic.Ac.). He may train further and obtain his bachelor's degree in acupuncture (B.Ac.); and finally his doctorate (Dr.Ac.). If the patient sees these certificates of qualification before treatment has begun he will know that he is in capable hands.

As a further safeguard there is in England a Register of Acupuncturists, and any student of the above college holding a Lic.Ac. or higher degree is eligible for nomination as a Member of the Register of Acupuncturists (M.R.Ac.) or as a Fellow (F.R.Ac.)

The Acupuncture Association is another establishment in England training to recognized standards. Its graduates will have letters similar to those above, followed by M.Ac.A. or F.Ac.A., Member or Fellow of the Acupuncture Association.

At the moment there is no such college in the United States that trains its students up to the standard required by the Chinese colleges. Even the conventional doctor who has certain qualifications in acupuncture may have received only a very short training.

One occasionally sees advertisements for acupuncture treatment. Can one rely on them?

It is stated quite clearly in the code of ethics that no registered or licenced practitioner may advertise at all. This bars anyone on the Register of Acupuncturists or any Member or Fellow of the Acupuncture Association from advertising.

The general public should be particularly wary of any form of advertising that indicates an unprofessional approach to medicine, such as door-to-door delivery of literature. There are commercial undertakings and clinics whose staff has not received recognized training or whose training has been inadequate.

Do you advocate receiving treatment from a practitioner who mixes acupuncture with another method of treatment?

Attempts have been made to westernize acupuncture and to bring it up to date by mixing it with other methods of treatment. It has, for example, been combined with electrical treatment, the electricity being used to stimulate the acupuncture points, and also with hypnotism, and so on. Some of these methods may get satisfactory results, but on the whole my advice would be for a prospective patient to find a practitioner who uses the traditional methods of acupuncture and who is fully trained according to Chinese standards.

15.

Acupuncture in the United States

Does a patient seeking acupuncture treatment in the United States today have much chance of finding a practitioner trained according to Chinese standards?

Unfortunately, just now there is little chance of doing so, but I believe the situation will greatly improve in the next few years. There is already a great deal of interest not only among the general public but also in the medical profession. Most people have now heard of acupuncture and know something about it. In particular, reports of operations performed under acupuncture anesthesia in Chinese hospitals are frequently in the news.

The medical profession in the United States has been open-minded, willing, and indeed anxious to study any new form of healing that comes its way. Acupuncture seems to be no exception. The fact that it is not yet more widely used is due rather to lack of reliable information and fully trained doctors of acupuncture to teach the subject than to any resistance to it.

Particular interest in certain aspects of acupuncture has been shown among medical men. They have been greatly impressed by the ability of a doctor of acupuncture to foretell the coming of disease in a patient before it has become manifest in the physical body. They have been impressed by Chinese methods of diagnosis and the fact that an experienced doctor of traditional Chinese acupuncture can often reveal more from reading the pulses than is shown by the most up-to-date medical equipment. They have been impressed by the power of acupuncture to heal or help in many cases where modern western medicine has failed. They are greatly interested in the possibility of operating while using acupuncture anesthesia on patients who would be unlikely to live through conventional anesthesia. They have been impressed by the help that acupuncture has been able to give in certain mental cases that have not responded to modern treatment.

Many American universities and medical schools are at this time trying to arrange courses in acupuncture, and there is a possibility of the establishment in the United States of a College of Chinese Acupuncture, provided that the legal problems of practicing acupuncture in the United States can be resolved. Public demand for this system of healing makes it essential that protection should be provided by the law to prevent the practice of acupuncture by anyone either unqualified or insufficiently qualified.

A large number of physicians and other qualified individuals have been sufficiently anxious to learn the principles and philosophy of traditional Chinese acupuncture and to train in its completely different methods of diagnosis to have undertaken study in these subjects. They are doing this despite their understanding that many years of study and experience will be needed before they can become fully proficient in this art. This speaks much for their enthusiasm and for the future of acupuncture in the United States.

Appendix: Effects of the Western Way of Life on Health

Earlier I mentioned that our western way of life places great strains and pressures upon us all, lowering our resistance to disease and leading to ill health. I left this statement unsupported because so much has already been written on the subject. However, as this whole question of our environment and way of life plays so vital a part in our general health, I feel it is most important to look at the evidence available as a whole, and to consider it from the viewpoint of its general effect on the health of us all.

I would say that there are three main ways in which western civilization is exposing all of us to situations that can only lead toward ill health.

First, we have a way of life that pursues an ever-higher standard of living. Our whole economy is geared to this. All the power of science and technology has been used to this end and has shaped our life-style. There is a general belief that wealth will bring happiness. In our anxiety to provide all men with material comforts, we have built up an environment that exposes mankind to a whole new area of problems and pressures.

Second, there is the rapid growth of population, which affects us both physically and mentally. There are the direct effects on the body of impure food, water, and air; and all of the pressure that is put upon us from trying to satisfy the needs of such vast numbers of people and from living in such close proximity to them.

Third, there is the arms and space race with its dominating influence in our society, resulting in exposure to still further dangers, pollution, and stresses.

The Pursuit of a High Standard of Living.

It is certainly true that we all like the comforts and conveniences that are made possible by a high standard of living. People want holidays abroad, color televisions, and the like. But we must consider the effects of a spiraling demand for a higher standard of living, and ask ourselves whether we can afford it. This demand for commodities must lead to bigger industry. And modern industry leads to pollution and stressful working conditions.

Industrial Pollution

We pour our poisons and wastes from factories into rivers, lakes, and seas. We discharge them into the air and bury them beneath the earth. We seal toxic waste into containers and dump it at sea. In transporting the raw materials and products we foul the air with exhaust fumes and the sea with used oil and sludge from our ships. There is no spot on this earth that remains unpolluted. The ecologists call constantly for immediate action. But the steady poisoning of our earth continues, spelling distress and death to one form of life after another.

Just think of some of the headline cases of recent years: crippling disease affecting hundreds of Japanese people due to mercury waste pouring from a factory into the sea and poisoning fish; containers of cyanide washed up on the beaches of Great

Britain, some of them leaking (one of the leading companies of the world regularly dumps cyanide waste in containers at sea); puffins in danger, whole colonies wiped out over the last year or two, believed to be due to the high levels of poisons from the paint and plastic industries that is contained in the algae on which they feed; and on and on.

Until recently we have felt that we cannot afford to deal satisfactorily with these dangerous side-effects of industry, for it would be very expensive to Western economy. Somehow we have tried to persuade ourselves that we, at all events, will not be affected. Other creatures and plants may be affected but man will escape unscathed.

It has become too expensive to repair or reuse articles and more and more things become disposable. The demand for raw materials, as it grows, becomes an enormous problem in itself, and the disposal of the rubbish created is an outsize problem resulting in more pollution.

Effects on Workers in Industry

A lively topic these days is job satisfaction. Few workers in industry seem to enjoy their work. Monotony is one of the big difficulties. And another is the shift system, in which workers are expected to be able to work, eat, and sleep at any time of the day or night.

This sort of thing places stress and strain on people, both physical and mental. As a result we have growing political and industrial unrest; strikes; slowdowns; demands for more pay, shorter hours, more holidays; and so on. When people are subjected to pressures year after year they very often get depressed and run down. And so they turn to props of one sort or another. We may drink too much, smoke too much, take drugs or pills of every description—stimulants, tranquilizers, sleeping pills, vitamin pills, indigestion pills, and headache pills.

People who are not getting satisfaction from their work will frequently look for enjoyment elsewhere. The result is a pleasure-seeking society with its consequent lowering of moral standards; debasing of sex; a lax attitude toward law and order; and a propensity for violence. Anarchy comes uncomfortably close.

Effects on the Individual

The drive for a higher standard of living seriously affects the individual. All too often the whole of a person's life is taken up with the acquisition of material things. He is tempted by a hundred and one attractively presented, skillfully advertised articles; and his desire to acquire them for himself and his family drives him along, very often making him unrealistically ambitious and leaving him no time to realize that he has been caught up in the rat race.

He rises from his bed, dashes to work, races home at night, eats a meal in front of the television, then goes to bed, to repeat the same thing the next day. He lavishes his time and affection on his car, his home, his furniture and his other possessions very often at the expense of his health. He is apparently prepared to sacrifice and abuse his body to achieve these ends.

Loss of Spiritual Life

Most important of all, in this hurly-burly and mad chase after the material comforts of life, man's spiritual needs are overlooked or pushed into the background. Scientific and technical knowledge tends to persuade us that there is no need for religion, for all that "myth and superstition," and we put our belief in the "isms" of humanism, realism, atheism, agnosticism.

It is my opinion that man's sickness will continue to increase until he stops seeking for his happiness in possessions and transitory pleasures.

Population Growth

The rise in population exposes our bodies and minds to many strains and stresses. Further industrialization follows the increased demand for food, water, housing, and all commodities and services, resulting in the sort of pollution and stresses already mentioned.

Production of Food

The increased demand for food has very far-reaching effects. The primary objective becomes quantity, not quality, and questionable methods are used to get the highest possible yield of crops and livestock. The land is saturated with chemical fertilizers. The runoff into waterways causes eutrophication, and slowly life in the water is killed and the river or lake becomes dead. Vegetables, fruit, and cereal grains are sprayed against pests and disease; many of the chemicals used are poisonous. Much of our meat and poultry comes from farms where the animals are kept in intensive units and have never lived in natural conditions, where they are fed on boosted foods and are filled with antibiotics and other drugs to prevent the diseases they become subject to under such conditions. These antibiotics and drugs pass into the milk, butter, cheese, and eggs that we eat. Water is needed in such large quantities that much is taken from polluted rivers and then has to be purified with such things as chlorine. Fluoride has to be added because we insist on feeding our children a diet guaranteed to cause tooth decay.

In order to feed the huge masses of people there are ever more convenience foods, pre-prepared, processed, and reconstituted foods, containing, as do many of the less obviously processed foods, all sorts of additives—artificial flavorings, colorings, and sweeteners; laboratory-made vitamins; preservatives; and such things, many of these proving to be carcenogenic (cancer-forming) after prolonged use.

We depend on the food we eat and the air we breathe to provide our bodies with their vital foods and to recharge our energy body, the Ch'i energy. Practically nothing that we eat today does not contain some unnatural substance or other, and no air that we breathe anywhere in the world is unpolluted. Thus our bodies are subjected to a constant strain. Some of the substances taken in may be toxic and some may not, but all have to be coped with by our bodies.

Air Pollution

Among the biggest causes of air pollution are the exhaust fumes of cars and other vehicles, and of course the increase in population has resulted in increased numbers of cars.

It would be relatively easy to remove the lead from the exhaust, one of its most dangerous constituents. Even at the North Pole the lead content of the air is now significant. Research on the continent of Europe shows that lead, along with carbon monoxide, has an insidiously harmful effect on city-dwellers, causing general malaise, headaches, depression, and fatigue.

The removal of carbon monoxide, which is harmful to all life, is a more difficult problem. Already in certain areas of California defoliation is advancing rapidly due to high levels of this gas. One method has been found (and unfortunately cars are actually in production that use this method) which considerably cuts down the quantities of carbon monoxide present in the exhaust, but results in the formation of high levels of nitrogen oxide. This, in time, affects the quality of the light reaching the surface of the earth. In this way, if it continues, we are gradually building up our own special screen of death!

Wastes

Ever-increasing amounts of sewage and detergent must be handled, much of which still goes straight into rivers and seas. Household rubbish is a headache in towns and cities. A particular problem is the large quantities of waste plastics that, if burned, give off toxic gases.

Loss of Countryside and Urbanization

More and more of our countryside is taken for town and road development and disappears under vast reservoirs. Increasing numbers of people find themselves living in sprawling urban areas, farther and farther removed from the open country, fresh air and space. A study of animals shows that the pressure of numbers creates a great deal of stress leading to irritability and fighting. Their normal behavioral patterns become completely upset. There is no reason to suppose that man behaves any differently when he is living in such close proximity to thousands of others.

Noise

Noise is an ever-increasing stress factor. Thousands of people are subjected daily to severe strain from living and working close to highways and airports. Our growing population demands mobility, and the resulting aircraft and traffic noise creates a serious health hazard. The continuous noise of towns and cities is the environment in which more and more people have to live.

The Arms Race and Space Race

Hazards of Pollution and Experiments

During the period of frequent nuclear testing, alarming effects were noted: levels of radioactivity in the atmosphere were rapidly becoming dangerous to life, fallout was found thousands of miles from the test sites, and very considerable disturbances were created in the atmosphere. High levels of fallout are occurring even from recent underground tests.

Many young people today, in contrast to earlier generations, run higher risks of bone cancer, leukemia, and thyroid troubles as a result of the 1950 nuclear tests. The enormous stockpiles of various weapons become obsolete from time to time and must be "disposed" of somewhere. It is chilling to remember the controversy that raged over the proposal by the U.S. Government to dump 27,000 tons of nerve gas in the Atlantic Ocean.

There is always the danger of something going wrong in experiments with modern methods of warfare. In Skull Valley, Utah, six thousand sheep died as a result of U.S. Army tests of the nerve gas, Vx. The threats of biological and chemical warfare are said to exceed by far even those of nuclear warfare. It was reported in *The Times* (July 4, 1969) that Gruinard, an island off the northwest coast of Scotland, was experimentally infected with anthrax. This proved so successful that it would be fatal for anyone to live there for probably up to a hundred years. On one occasion scientists from all over the world warned the United States of the possibly irreparable danger of putting a vast quantity of "needles" into space for some military research project. The United States military advisers chose to ignore these warnings and urged approval of the scheme. The "needles" went up.

It seems shortsighted in the extreme that the fears one nation has of another should prompt it to act in such a way as to endanger the balance of life on this earth, and the balance of the earth in relation to the cosmos. Little is known of the consequences on the biosphere and stratosphere of many of our arms race and space race experiments.

Effects on Mental Health

The arms race has had a hard-to-measure yet real effect on the mentality of young people. Overpowered by the pointlessness of living, great numbers of students have suffered in the past years from depression, lethargy, and fear. Others have become militant and anarchistic in their determination to break down the structure of the society that has led to the arms race.

Acknowledgment

The author has found two publications of particular help in the preparation of this book: the writings of Sheila Ostrander and Lynn Schroeder, and of Professor Kim Bong Han, to which reference has been made in the text. He expresses his indebtedness to them.

73 74 75 76 77 10 9 8 7 6 5